MY TBI: MOVE FORWARD WITH HOPE

BETSY L. DUVAL

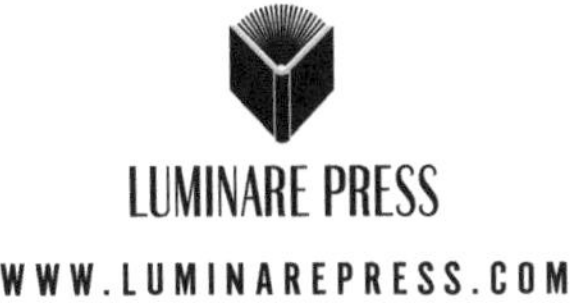

LUMINARE PRESS

WWW.LUMINAREPRESS.COM

My TBI: Move Forward with Hope
© Betsy L. Duval

Printed in the United States of America

Cover Art: Betsy L. Duval

Luminare Press
467 W 17th Ave
Eugene, OR 97401
www.luminarepress.com

LCCN: 2016944047
ISBN: 978-1-944733-01-8

Also by Betsy L. Duval
My TBI Journey, lulu.com

Dedication

This book is dedicated to my extended family, friends,

and TBI support group

Contents

My Purpose 1

New Day 3

Survive to Thrive 6

Independence 12

Close Encounters 14

Doctors and Pills 18

Thought list 20

Staying yourself 22

My Jims 24

Forward progress 29

Cabin and Transportation 32

St. Teresa 36

TBI Support Group 40

Professions 43

Predestination 45

Forward Therapy 54

Hugs and HOPE 60

Additional TBI Resources 63

My Purpose

Hopefully I will be able to convey to you the feelings that have come to me going through this journey. There are quite a few people who are going on the journey with me and we'll be here together for the rest of our lives. Some of them I never knew before but, like you, became connected when they realized how much is involved in how all of our brains function. This is something most of us don't even consider. It just works the way it is supposed to. Why think about it?

This is not to be about me. I hope it includes you and can give you guidance and help.

We all function with HOPE. Hope that what I am cooking will come out tasting all right. Hope you will get there safely. Hope that what I smell isn't something on fire. Every day, in everything we do there is some kind of hope.

When we wake up in the morning we need hope. We need to give it to each other.

I'm writing this to honor those who were there for me.

Chapter 1

New Day

I don't know if you read my first and continuing journey, "My TBI Journey, Stay on the Train". Maybe you can still get a copy.

A few minutes ago I was sitting on the back porch. I had been sleeping lightly and around four o'clock the lightning and thunder came on suddenly and I started thinking.

In 30 days it will be exactly three years since the wreck occurred. I don't want this to sound dramatic so I'll just say I received a TBI (traumatic brain injury).

Sitting on the porch with beads in my hands, candle lit, and a cup of coffee next to me, I was analyzing how grateful I am to have come so far. Hope that next Wednesday I will have the chance to make another step forward in coming out of this. I know it will never be the same. Not "perfect". But maybe perfect is not what I am looking for. Right now what I still can't do is make my mind and vision coordinate with each other so that I instantly can focus correctly on something. It might have something to do with the muscles that hold the eye in place. That is evidently new as far as rehabilitation therapy is concerned. Wednesday is going to be my appointment for evaluation.

This morning when I woke up it was lightning. I could see it and possibly feel it in my mind. When I said something to Jim it was hard for me to talk. I could talk but it was some slight kind of an effort. Maybe it had something to do with the electricity. I've never been afraid of lightning or thunder so I don't think it has to do with fear. Maybe the nerves stimulated in the brain have something to do with it. This same slight difficulty in talking has happened to me before but I don't think it was while it was raining. I'll try to keep a note of it when it happens again.

For those of you who read my first book, you know how my waking up in the morning effects my day. It's how I get connected physically and emotionally to what I plan on doing that day. Hope to be able to adjust calmly to the changes that come. I've learned that fighting changes are out of your hands. Getting strongly, emotionally upset takes a lot of negative energy. I try to handle things as positively as possible.

　　　　Betsy L. Duval

Just to let you know. When you are reading this if something is not spelled right, not indented as it should be, not the same size etc. it is because I am using it just as it was given to me by someone, or it shows how my mind is still developing.

Chapter 2

Survive to Thrive

When I was life-flighted to TMH emergency room I received a treatment. Since I don't even know how to describe it, I will let Dr. Jake (the creator) tell you about it in his own words:

It was August 5th, 1995. It was an exciting time and a proud time as my older brother had been accepted into Medical School at the University of Florida and a tight group of seven friends including myself were moving him down to Gainesville for the weekend before he got started. We were all at a restaurant on the second night, a Saturday. After playing a sober game or two of darts the whole gang was ready to head home for some much needed rest as we had laid out late the night before. I headed to the restroom on the way out and was the last of my buddies to exit the building. That's the last thing I remember. To hear the story later a very large man, a vagrant, blindsided me with a punch in the left jaw. I fell straight down and hit my head on the curb. I would find out, 24 hours later, that the assault had resulted in three hemorrhages in my brain. I went to the hospital that night but was not given a CT scan yet, told to leave and I would be fine. I slept on the floor of the apartment unfortunately off and on for the next 18 hours. Everybody drove home but me and my brother of course as I wasn't feeling well. My brother had engagements in preparation for the start of classes so I was in the apartment alone that next evening. My head was by the phone and I heard it ring. It was my dad checking on us. By the time of the call my brain had swelled so much on the left side that I had lost proper function of my speech center. Thankfully, my father recognized my slurred speech and called a friend. The friend broke into the apartment through the window and took me to the hospital to get a CT scan. This CT scan showed three hemorrhages in my brain as I had only an hour or two to live. The doctors put me on an experimental drug called Decadron; it was a steroid that reduced inflammation and it worked miraculously. I stayed in the ICU for 8 to 10 days and was in and out of consciousness. I was finally able to get up and try walking again. Once I was able to walk far enough to get to the elevator, I was good enough to go home. I started physical therapy school about a month later but I still had some amnesia from the accident. I could not drive so my mother and grandmother would drive me everywhere, including school. I made it through class, but it was difficult because my memorization was not where it used to be. I lost my sense of smell from the brain injury. It cut my olfactory nerves and for a while the headaches were excruciating.

About 15 months later I was at the neurosurgeon getting a check-up, but the short- term amnesia was still driving me crazy. The doctor said that this normally takes about 18 months to come back, and if it didn't I may just be stuck with what I had left. Then one day, I woke up a couple months later and I just knew everything was back to normal. My memory was back. So I moved forward with my physical therapy degree and concentrated on neuro-physical therapy.

I worked for two and half years with neurologically impaired children with brain injuries in and around the time of birth; cerebral palsy and hemorrhages to name a few. I then took an outpatient job with all the kids who had neurological impairments. A special patient named Tyler had a unique effect on me. We taught him how to walk at age 3 before he passed away with AIDS.

Now I was ready to try my hand at research so I decided to go back for my Ph.D. in Neuroscience and focus Translational Medicine. This was partially because I wanted to help kids like Tyler and a lot because I just love the brain. Translational medicine is a discipline within biomedical and public health research that aims to improve the health of individuals and the community by "translating" bench-science findings into diagnostic tools, medicines, procedures, policies and education.

I was accepted into the Neuroscience Program in August of 1999 at Florida State University. This program had three departments associated with it, Psychology, Biology and the Department of Nutrition, Food, and Exercise Sciences. My principal

    Betsy L. Duval

investigator was Cathy Levenson who had a PhD in Biomedical Sciences and Nutrition. The major focus of her lab was to look at trace metals in neurodegenerative disorders. These models mimicked Alzheimer's and Parkinson's disease. We looked at models of how the nerves were actually dying and what we could do to protect them. It took me four years to complete my PhD.

Within the last year and a half, my work was focused on micro-array where we looked at gene expression in conditions where it was altered from depression and anxiety. Specifically, we looked at the hippocampus where the memory centers are and looked at the olfactory bulb which ties into depression and anxiety in Parkinson's and Alzheimer's disease. My PhD thesis was on the role that trace metals had in neuronal gene expression. I did however along the way have authorship on a paper that used a penetrating traumatic brain injury model to evaluate the role of zinc as a neuroprotectant.

Being personally connected to brain injury and now having a PhD to do drug development via translational medicine in the neurosciences, I decided to do a post-doctoral fellowship at Emory University in Atlanta working with Donald Stein, Ph.D. and David Wright, M.D. I worked there for eight to ten months as a postdoctoral student and then got promoted to assistant director of the Brain Research Lab, the largest lab in the Department of Emergency Medicine.

We studied the mechanisms in which progesterone worked and its effects in treating moderate to severe brain injuries in animals. Plus, we looked at clinical blood samples that were coming out of the use of progesterone in brain injured humans. Most of these patients came into the hospital in a coma. The ProTECT trial was must first glimpse into Drug Development, Clinical Trials and understanding the FDA.

In the fall of 2006 I returned home and took a job as a Course Director at the Florida State University College of Medicine. I very much enjoyed teaching but my passion for translational medicine continued. In 2011 we created the first drug and patents for concussion treatment. From here, in June of 2012, we incorporated a Drug Development Company, Prevacus.

I am proud to say that we are now approved for human trials using our drug, PRV-002 for concussion. As a lightweight nasal spray we will be able to get our drug acutely to field of play, battle and emergency vehicles. The drug is 380-fold safe and we are able to get over 4-fold more to the brain than other delivery devices. We hope to have this drug FDA approved within the next 3 years. Recently, we have started a new drug project targeting pathologies associated with Alzheimer's and Chronic Traumatic Encephalopathy.

My recovery was a blessing. Most people with the severe nature of head trauma and bleeding on the brain that I experienced are permanently disabled both physically and cognitively. I'm glad I embraced my brain injury and I'm trying to help others that were not as fortunate as I was. My mom calls me every August 5th to wish me

　　　　Betsy L. Duval

Happy Anniversary for my survival date. She told me this past Christmas that she can rest in peace now knowing why God spared my life.

—Jacob W. Van Landingham

That's what got me slowly going again. I'm still going strong.

Chapter 3

Independence

Again, to those who read my first and continual journey about my TBI, you know how strongly our boys and Jim were in my recovery. Presently Scott, our oldest, is halfway around the world with Ginger and our grandkids. Jay is so far away in the U.S. with Amy and our other grandkids that we have to go by plane. Ben is just a few hours away by car. We have good, strong connections with all of them.

Bekah moved from Michigan last year to be a few blocks around the corner from us. She and I do girl shopping and get our nails done without any guys tagging along. Since I probably will not be able to drive again, it is super to have somebody else who offers to drive me places.

That has turned out to be the most frustrating part of this independence thing. I use to drive all the way to our cabin in the North Georgia mountains by myself and spend time up there with friends. There it is an entirely different environment. It has to be frustrating for Jim to have to handle me when all I want to do is needle him jokingly. I've tried to ride a three-wheel bike or drive a golf cart, wanting to go three blocks to Publix or three blocks the other way to TJ Maxx. We haven't been able to handle that yet.

Presently Jim might give a golf lesson or play a couple of rounds a week with old friends. He definitely doesn't worry about me being okay. He still keeps his cell phone on all the time and can hang around with the guys and get away from me. That and being able to give lessons around the corner is where his heart is. The weekly golf tournament on T.V. is where he spends his T.V. time. That isn't my choice so I go in a quiet space and write, paint, or read.

Chapter 4

Close Encounters

We have three boys Scott, Jay, and Ben. We moved here thirty years ago. Jim is a PGA professional and our move got him in touch with quite a few of the locals. Many of them were also golfers and all became close friends. Venice was a small town with local residence year around. All of our kids grew up together. If something was going on at your house everyone would know about it. If you were out of town and your kids weren't where they were supposed to be you would know.

We are annually supported by the "snow birds" that flock here for the winter months. That's what keeps the whole place going financially and culturally. They come here from all over. From Canada, the northern states, and even our southern cousins come because the weather is usually so perfect.

I started walking with a close neighbor who had girls our son's ages. We walked most every morning before going to work. At that time I was the director of the infant/toddler pre-school at our church. Another neighbor started walking with us and eventually we, along with our friends, formed a book club. We all became very close while we were dealing with kids, their school activities, sports etc. Some have since past on and others joined us. But some of the original of us are still together.

The reason that I included this chapter is to let you know how neat it is that we all have somebody that we are connected to that make a difference in our lives even though we don't realize it at the time. We just live it.

February the book club is coming here to my house for lunch. I chose the book we read this last month. We are all close, and have been through a lot all these years. It is a challenge for me now to be able to count out who will be here. Where are the plates I am going to use? What recipe is needed and how am I going to make it all work? It's a real challenge.

Scott, our oldest son, came in Wednesday. He's leaving on Sunday, which is the day the girls are coming for lunch. I need a list of groceries, be able to go in Publix and find what I need with help, set the table right etc. Tomorrow I mix up what I'm cooking. What time do I put it on before they come? All of this I did before not even thinking about it or stressing out. Keep calm!!! It will all work out.

It did all work out. Now just being able to do all of it myself felt real good. It's another step forward.

This is March and I just had lunch with my book club friends. I invited any who wanted to contribute something to you to do it here. One in particular who has been real close to me through it all can tell you how difficult it is to deal with someone who has had a TBI.

The accident happened November the 3rd. My friend Carol was sorting through some old things and came up with something she found that she wrote when she and Don came to TMH where I was, 300 miles away. When you read this you will know I have definitely come out way better than the doctors ever thought would be possible.

Here is her story:

Wed, Nov 16. Drove to Tallahassee to visit Betsy. Scott & Jim met us outside the Specialty Select Rehab. Scott took us inside and prepared us.

Betsy's face looked perfect, no cuts or bruises, (a miracle). Her eyes are closed. She is being monitored for BP, heart rate, oxygen. She has no tubes now.

She moans at times, throws her right leg around like she is doing yoga. She has a very tight grip on her hands.

Jim, Scott & Bob Duval (Jim's brother) met with

    Betsy L. Duval

Betsy's two Drs.Today, Nov 17.

Jim's hope is to have her in a facility as soon as possible in Sarasota. She will probably be there for at least six months with kickass therapy before being sent home.

Dr. said he will have his wife back and his boys their Mom, but not as she was a month ago. She will retain what she knew but will not be able to learn anything new.

The CAT scan was better than the 1st that was done. No more bleeding in the brain. The left side is not moving. The right side is active. She will walk, probably with a walker. Pray that her eyes open. Her sight is questionable.

Chapter 5

Doctors and Pills

When I first came back from TMH after more than four months I had seen more than eight doctors, a good number of nurses and rehabilitation specialists. At that time I was on nine different medications and my daily and weekly pillbox was totally full. Someone else had to make sure I took it at the right time. Gradually I was weaned off of all the medication.

Four weeks ago I took my last natural pill that gives me what my body naturally produces to help my brain relax and easily fall asleep. That was another step forward. Me feeling like I could count on the fact that my body had progressed to the point that I could sleep long enough and wake up naturally again. I didn't have to have a doctor decide that for me. At this point all I am taking are salt, fish oil and multivitamins.

I have an appointment tomorrow with my neuro-ophthalmologist who may be the last doctor who I need to deal with that is involved with what happened to me in the wreck. It will feel good for me to be able to tell him that I feel like I have reached the full extent of my recovery.

When I saw him he asked me what I needed to make sure of when I rode my new bike. When I shrugged my shoulders he said, "We don't need another injured head. Make sure you wear your helmet"

Chapter 6

Thought list

*W*hen you think of something write it down. Do it if you can. Tell it to somebody. Don't try to keep it in your memory. If you do you'll regret that you didn't do any of it. It's no good to say, "I meant to do it but forgot".

If I think of something, I might be doing something else, and when I walk out of the room I'm saying to myself a certain sentence and it takes time to remember why I am saying it. Example: "I should have gone there before here". Where is there and why? Cut that article out before it gets thrown away.

When I first was getting my memory back I had post-it tags in different places. On the refrigerator, in the computer room, under the telephone, plus. Eventually I was able to put them together plus other notes and write my first book. They are presently using it at TMH in the rehab for families or people who have gone through the same things we did.

Now when I write a post-it note it at least gets to be next to all the others I write and it doesn't get lost in different places on the floor.

This same thing happens to quite a few people. Maybe it's natural but mine has not been natural. Thank goodness I'm finally able to keep it straight.

Chapter 7

Staying yourself

I just read in the stack of stuff piled on my desk, in some sort of order, an e-mail that came in while I was "out of it". It was from a close friend of mine who I grew up with. My younger sister Tricia kept everybody in touch with how things were going with me on Caringbridge.com. This friend and I were born four days apart in the same hospital in Tallahassee. She is one of my core friends whose profession is working with people who have had TBIs, strokes, etc. that have affected their brain.

The message on the e-mail told those who were there working with me, Jim and the boys etc., to make sure they didn't steer me in the wrong direction. Don't try to make me into someone I'm not. Since I could not remember how I felt about certain things but just reacted for reasons I didn't remember, they should let me sort it out in my own mind. Let my personality come back through. Don't try to

 Betsy L. Duval

explain to me why I feel that way.

For example: We had a close relationship with a couple who were married when we all were younger. They went through a very difficult personal tragedy and while dealing with it one of them died. We were all very close. Within a short time the survivor remarried. After all of this happened with me with the wreck, I personally tried to make sure I quietly didn't bring attention to myself and "played nice". Needless to say it took particular personal strength when Jim and I spent a night at their house to "play nice". I finally figured out why I felt so negative in that situation. The last time we saw them I was told "You are nicer to be around than you use to be". For that I get a gold star. My true feelings I now know are okay. I'm able to become myself.

Where am I going from here? I've become a partial autobiographer. I was able to re-teach myself how to create artistically. I was an art teacher. I was a legal guardian for the elderly with at least four clients when the wreck happened. I was told the other day the fact that I can both focus on writing, and painting at the same time tells me that both sides of my brain are working like it is supposed to.

What I deal with every morning when I wake up is "How am I going to get through the day". Make sure not to focus on the negative possibilities but hope for the positives. Something good will come your way.

Chapter 8

My Jims

"Jim" is a special name for me. There are many of them in my life. On the top of my list is my attachment to the one I have been with now for 48 years. That's the one who has put up with me and all of my stuff. We just went to our cabin in the Georgia mountains and celebrated our anniversary there with the deer, turkey, baby geese etc. It is a totally different quiet, soothing, peaceful environment.

Another Jim is one who came along when we moved to Venice and he grew up with the boys. He spent many nights here and calls himself our number 4.

The third to come along has helped me get my ability to re-learn how to write and get my feelings out to you. He is also very special to me. He had self-published a small book that we had a copy of in our coffee table in Venice. When I "came back" and was looking through things on the table it slowly came to me (that's how things come to me now, SLOWLY) that I could use what I had put down on paper in my notebook, what other people had written about their feelings and involvement with me, and put it in a self-published book. I really didn't want anything changed or edited. Hopefully it would show how I had slowly progressed to be able to write full sentences and spell the words right. Since this Jim had done this himself before, I felt like this could be the way to go. I am also an artist so writing about this and my struggle to get back to being able to mix colors , physically use brushes, see well enough to detail what I wanted to, and express my emotions that way, was a forward improvement goal for me.

In my first book I took one of my paintings of St. Teresa (my family cottage on the Gulf of Mexico when I grew up) to show what I as originally able to do before the accident happened, and used a print of it.

This Jim helped me understand how I could use all of this to get my first book self-published. Just to let you know, when an accident like this happens and it affects your brain, it is almost impossible to multi-task. That means if you have an idea, say go in the bedroom and put on your shoes, and you walk through the family room and the T.V. is on, you stop in the middle of the room hearing it, and then can't remember where you were going before and for what.

It basically required me to be able to finish writing my first book and get it published, before I dared try to start re-learning how to be an artist. No multitasking.

SUCCESS. I published my first book, which they are now using copies of at TMH to help their rehabilitation staff let families read, and talk about. Families who have gone through what my family and I are going through.

Since that was published I have been able to go back to learning to be an artist. The picture here shows you how successful I've been. I have another painting in progress while I'm writing. This lets me know I'm going to be able to concentrate on two things at once again. That is definite forward progress.

Let's get back to my number one Jim. I was raised in the south with, "Yes Mam, no Sir, bless her heart". When my mouth opens and my hands start moving you definitely know where I come from. I feel that every one of us is born with a talent. Hopefully each one gets to use it eventually throughout our lives here and it makes us happy. Example: cook (chef), building (contractor).

My Jim grew up and felt the desire to play and become a golf pro. His dad was a pro and it has gone throughout his family. That, and the fact that he was born and raised in the north. What was the likelihood that we would meet and spend forty-eight plus years together still going strong? There are no coincidences. It's all predestined. Before the wreck happened we both had our lives going strong and independent. Me coming from teaching art in schools, directing an infant/toddler/pre-school, becoming a licensed guardian for the elderly or disabled, and Jim very successfully putting full time into teaching, playing in tournaments, and making golf his focus.

The accident totally changed this. No more independence for either of us. A shock. Twenty four seven it was all about me. First I had to learn how to move anything and get it to work right. Jim was there right beside me so I could touch him and know he was there. That is predestination.

We've been "coming back" for three and a half years now and this sounds strange but I feel there was a definite reason for my wreck in our life together. It has definitely brought us closer. We have learned that sharing our feelings about things is more important than arguing or anger. We keep in closer touch with family and friends and reach out to make new friends. We never know how many people we touched before until they all came to help us physically, emotionally and with prayers. Never leave someone without a hug. You never know if it's going to be the last time.

Jim is stuck with me permanently. "Bless his heart". Since I won't be able to drive again he's my transportation. At least he gets to socialize on his own without me tagging along and we can go out together with friends. He can go out and give lessons or play a round with friends and then have a drink at the bar and not worry about me. That gives me time to independently concentrate on my art work. That is a plus for both of us.

    Betsy L. Duval

Chapter 9

Forward progress

Progress!! That is what is important. You need to keep making positive progress. Sometimes it is hard to stay positive. Once I was able to finish my first TBI Journey, and get it self-published, that was great. I felt I would then be able to concentrate and again focus on re-learning how to draw and paint. That is my profession and talent.

I need to teach myself how to mix colors, what colors to use where, how to stroke the brush, what size, shape and texture of brush to use, what media (oil or acrylic), how to clean everything up. I was an art teacher and had to recall it all.

It took me about two months to gradually pick a canvas, draw a manatee and Kemp Ridley turtle hugging each other, choose oil paints and brushes and slowly figure out how I was going to create that feeling.

I was on the last legs of getting it done when I

got a call from someone who knew what I had gone through. Since I was an artist she wondered if I had a picture that I could possibly let her use for an exhibit that was going to be in three weeks. I had to think fast. What would it take to finish this picture? Waves, clouds, sky, sunlight, etc. How long would it take for the canvas to dry? I'm calling it "Buddies."

Needless to say I hurried up on it and found what I needed and made up the rest. I finished it in record time but that was all I had to focus on. I feel like I can again concentrate and become involved for hours with no interruptions. My vision has improved so that I can pick out the details I need to express what I want.

It's finished now and will be ready to go, and dry, in a week and a half. It's another wonderful thing that I accomplished on my bucket list. The end of this chapter just happened. This is Tuesday morning.

Last Friday I took the finished and dried painting to be exhibited. Going in I was surprised and excited at how many artists we had at St. Marks. There were quilters, sculptors, potters, printers etc. One of my original clay pieces of Madonna and child and my TBI book were put with my painting on display. It felt good to again be recognized for my talent. More of my "coming out" completed.

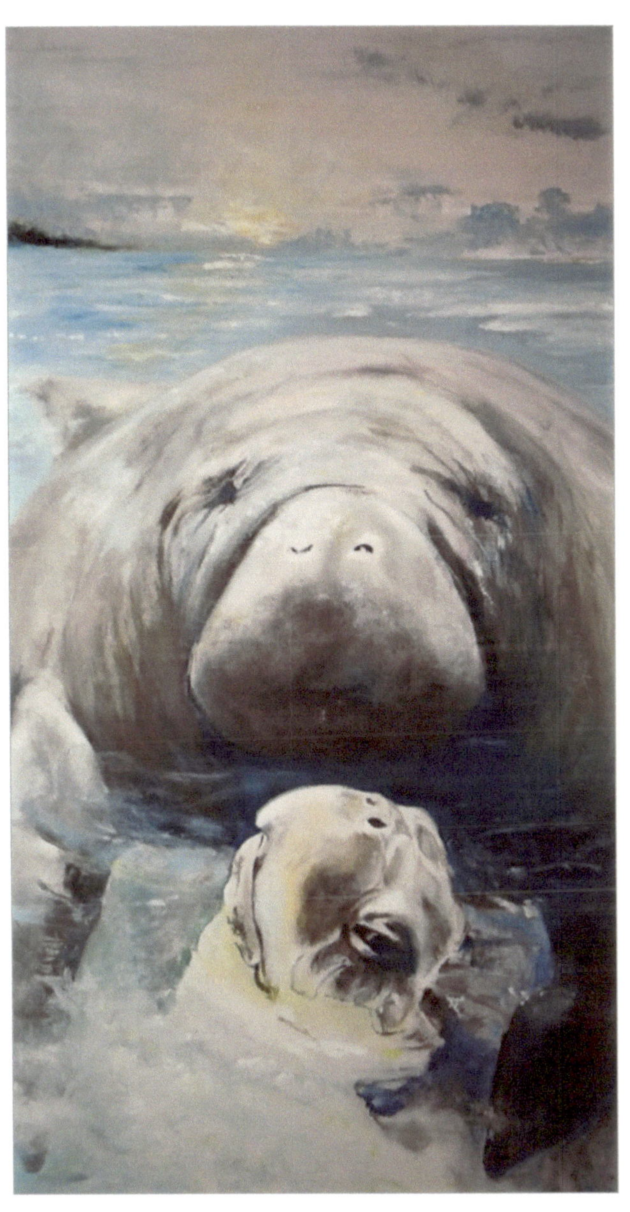

Chapter 10

Cabin and Transportation

What about Transportation? I lost my independence. I could get in the car at eight in the morning, stop for lunch, roadside park mid-afternoon, and be at our northeast Georgia cabin in the mountains by eight that night. There is no T.V. here, only a radio. Deer have a path morning and night through the woods in the front yard and up the side of the cabin eating the lilies in the spring. The bear pry open the lid on the garbage can, which is bungee corded shut. The geese call on the pond. A different world is here.

The cabin is a special place for Jim and me. It is our quiet world. I get up and light my candle by the pond. The bullfrog gives his low wake up croak, crickets start their buzzing, birds start their identifying calls. If it's still quiet, the wild turkeys

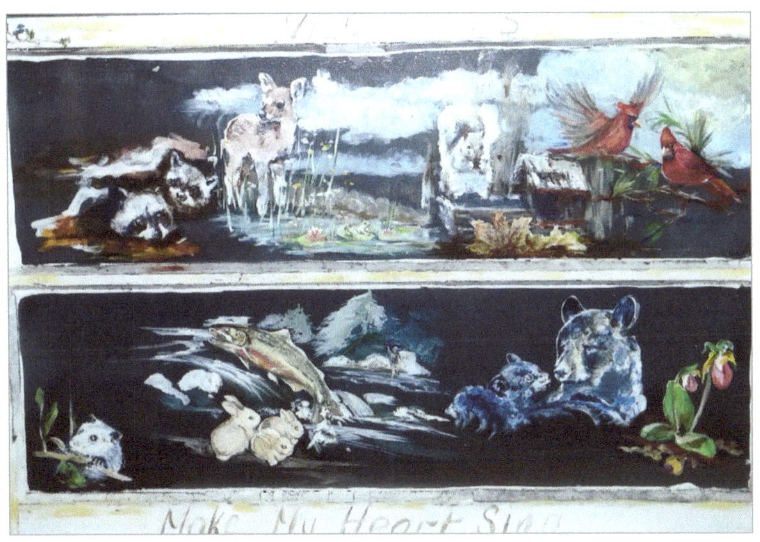

Wild things make my heart sing

start their slow trek through the brush in the woods. There is nothing like it. It gives you a special quiet soul feeling.

For me now driving a car is no more. Then I thought, "If not a car now, a golf cart would do". That would be easy. Would it be gas or electric? Do you have to use a seat belt on the road? What about a license? Can I renew my license on my birthday? What does it take to renew my license? Well at least let's look at one. There's the lot selling them and there's one that is street legal with a Florida tag. Let's try it out. Okay, what do I punch or shift to back it up? This is harder than I thought. Gas? Brake? Where is the blinker for the turn signal?

If we were actually on the road I would have to be

looking where the cars were, lights changing, make sure we stayed in the right lane. Oh, my! This could be dangerous. Not an option. Ben, Scott and Jay were against that anyway. Jim didn't voice his opinion even though he was in the cart with me while I was doing the driving.

The more, deeper, desire was just to get out of the driveway by myself. Look! There's a couple and each have a tricycle and hers' has a basket. Maybe I could do that and eventually go 5 blocks to TJ Maxx or if I'm really careful 5 blocks across the highway to Publix. Publix would be less of a desire.

"Can I help you?" I just want to try one out. "Just turn the handle, don't lean like you do on a regular bike."—"How does that feel?"—"Yeah, we can lower the handle bar and adjust the level of the seat."—"Yeah we can deliver it. It will be an extra $25.00."

"Betsy, maybe we need to talk to the boys about this." "This is my decision and I'm paying for it—period." A pretty green color.

Okay, now out of the garage making sure the flag doesn't catch in the door. My, I didn't realize how steep the driveway is. Wait till I have to peddle back up it. Guess I have to put the break on, get off and push it up and back into the garage. Acquiring even outdoor independence is a challenge.

Step two onto the street and around the small block. I ride the bike and Jim is walking behind with Maddie, our little fluffy white rescue. Stay on the right side and around that car parked in the road.

Step three, day three around the big block with Maddie on a pillow in the basket with Jim following.

Step four, me putting Maddie in the basket myself and going around the small block alone.

I'm slowly making my TJ Maxx dream come true. Maybe not making it to our Georgia cabin alone but settling for a TJ Maxx without Jim worrying about me.

I always promise him I won't do anything that he isn't comfortable with.

Chapter 11

St. Teresa

Jim asked me what I wanted for my birthday this year. I didn't even hesitate. Nothing materialistic would do. It had to be "special". The ultimate feeling. I'm writing this early in the morning. The clocks moved forward yesterday morning.

Day before yesterday was my birthday. I'm not going to relate to you how old I am. I have on my flannel P-Js and robe, socks and slippers. We're at St. Teresa, my "Island in the Sun". I'm sitting in a rocking chair on the front porch looking out over the water.

Our cottage is a fourth generation hand-me-down on the Gulf of Mexico. It is forty-five minutes south of Tallahassee. I was born and raised in Tallahassee and spent a lot of my summer every year here. We were raised with rowboats, ski boats, slaloms, fishing poles, oyster tongues, crab traps, seine nets, scallop buckets, etc.

Here it was always an escape from the noise. There were no T.V.s and no confusion about the rules. A mandatory hour or more after lunch was nap time. No matter how many were in the cottage there was no talking. As kids we had to make sure we went to the bathroom before bed as there wasn't even walking on the floor after that time. When you got in bed my grandma had us sit on the side so she could wash our feet. We didn't want to sleep on sandy sheets.

Now the whole area is called the "Forgotten Coast" and most of us want to keep it that way.

During the Second World War the beach was used to train troops to use amphibian ducts to come ashore. When we grew up the hollowed out ditches ran along the side of the dock that is still kept there. Behind the cottages on the other side of highway 98 was the landing strip of the area teaching the pilots to fly in and out, over the water, etc. When I grew up the barracks for the troops had become summer camp cottages for the Episcopal Church kids. It was originally called Camp Gordan Johnson and then became Camp Weed. Us local kids always were jealous that those kids had more privileges than we did. None of us realized how blessed we all were.

My granddaddy and his brother owned a drug store in Tallahassee, Fain Drug Company. The bank was Lewis State Bank. The doctors, lawyers, and Indian chiefs each had bought a cottage on the gulf and when the war came they were taken over by the government. Over my head now on the wall hangs a sign with a duck in a rowboat over waves. It says "NAVIGATION SCHOOL". That was outside our cottage. Evidently each cottage was used for something. Some for officers' quarters, etc. When the war was over the cottages went back to the owners.

Mom and Dad had three girls, no boys. My older sister Margie was in the wreck with me. My younger sister Tricia came every day to TMH for over three months to stay with me when I was in rehab. They and their husbands were here with Jim and I for my birthday, day before yesterday. That was my birthday gift from Jim and all of them. Very special.

Since we all grew up down here and all were raised in Tallahassee, all of the cottages are still owned by descendants of the original owners. Every time any of us comes here, whoever is on the beach or sidewalk going to the dock, owned by all of us, is usually kin to somebody we know. If it's warm enough, and somebody is sitting on their porch in a rocking chair, you stop to talk to them. That's the southern way. No strangers allowed. There are maybe eighteen cottages along this stretch. It is called the "Old St. Teresa". Around the corner and down the beach is presently referred to as St. Teresa but nothing here is commercial. Blessed.

I'm in the same chair here this morning. It's 4:30 A.M. This is the hardest day for me as we are leaving. When the car pulls out of the gate it means it will be

     Betsy L. Duval

a long time before I will be able to sit on the front porch in the rocking chair, light my candle, quietly hear the waves come in and watch the sun come up over the water. Another day and we're blessed to be here.

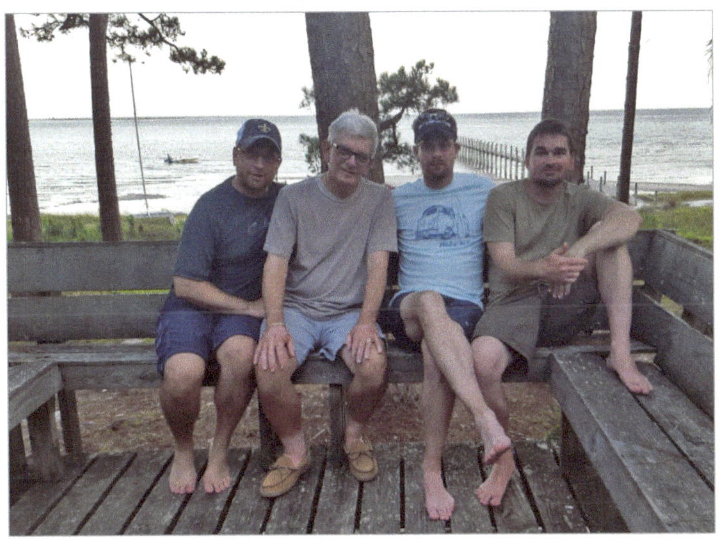

Jim and the boys at St. Teresa

Chapter 12

TBI Support Group

I woke up this morning. It was early to get up. If I'm fully awake there is no way I can turn over and go back to sleep. At that point I either lie there and plan my whole day and try to decide what I am going to put on to wear, so I will look like I'm ready to go grocery shopping, to the gym, to church…. Maybe if I've been in bed awake for a long time I reluctantly get up and turn on the coffee, go get the paper then quietly read the news. This morning I was thinking so fast I just had to get up and write it down.

Those of us who have had a TBI, stroke, spinal injury etc. go once a month to a meeting together as a support group. We share with each other what we have gone through and are going through. It's something that never stops for any of us and we all have different challenges. Some of us have similar things we deal with. Some of us have gone through things and have come out of them so can help others know how we dealt with them. The name of our group is the "Suncoast Center for Independent Living".

There are no doctors who have a degree in helping you solve this. If there were, for most of us, there is no way to make enough money to even pay for an appointment. Our injuries are both physical and mental and there is no "cure". For some of us we have gotten far enough so that we can dress ourselves, eat at the table, walk straight, talk, and we do most of the things everybody else does. For most of us you cannot see anything different about us if you didn't know us.

The first time Jim and I went to a meeting I came out thinking "I can belong to this club and be a real member. I don't have to prove anything to anybody to get in and they all accept me". Luck again showed its head. That is a really good feeling. But you don't really want to be a member of this club.

I'm not an oddball. The problem I thought about when I woke up this morning early was "How many more of us are out there that don't have any idea of where to go. Is there some way we could all get together somewhere and make enough money to help us all get through?" I'm lucky enough to have the boys and Jim but some have nobody to help them. Is there some way we could all get together and contribute something we have the talent for?

I was getting discouraged. Was this all the way I

was going to be able to get it going again? Was this how I was going to be for the rest of my life? Was I going to walk this way, think this way, sees this way, feel this way?

"Challenged". That's the word I've been looking for. Even if you are challenged to do something, it might not be possible to accomplish it because something has been damaged.

Every once in a while I just want to sit down and cry but don't dwell on it because I know that dwelling on it just makes it worse. I know that my vision has a tremendous effect on everything I do every day. I think I have hoped that by doing these eye exercises every day it will gradually make things come out all right. It will never be perfect again, but what is perfect? I think my problem is: How will I know when I have gone as far as I am able to go with the damage that occurred to my head? Jim still isn't comfortable with the term "damaged brain".

How will I know??? I think there is no way anybody else would be able to tell you that that is as far as you can hope to go. At some point do you just accept that you will be this way for the rest of your life and just live with it? I think everyone of us in our support group is "challenged" by this every day.

We are all in a personal battle and thankfully have the support of others who are going through their own battle. There I've written it down and gotten it out of my head and onto paper. What's next??

     Betsy L. Duval

Chapter 13

Professions

The hardest thing for me when I finally sorted everything out was my profession. I was a licensed professional guardian. That meant I had charge of where the person lived, who they lived with, if they were comfortable with the person or people they were with every day and if they were happy there. What did they bring into the guardianship with me? They brought their possessions, finances, relatives, lawyers etc. Basically I felt the need to make sure their life worked out the best that it could.

There were at least four clients that I had when the wreck happened. That meant I tried to see them and spend an hour or more with them every week. One was in an apartment with her caregiver, another in an assisted living and I would go have lunch with her. She was an ice cream lover and I would take her out for fresh made Ice cream at a local shop. One could count on me picking him up and dropping him off to have coffee with his friend while I went shopping nearby for an hour. I was very close with all of them.

What was I going to do now? They needed somebody to take care of them and it couldn't be me. I think we all have divine connections. How do I handle this? A close lawyer friend approached. I was able to hand the list over to him and he blessed me with the willingness to handle it all. Evidently I had it all in a file in some kind of order. I can't even tell you now where it was or how I had it.

I haven't been able yet to make contact with any of them. That is one thing I haven't figured out how to handle. I'm afraid I would just look at one of them and start to cry. I do a lot of that these days. I found out yesterday that one of them had died. That is very hard.

This is on my bucket list.

Chapter 14

Predestination

I've said this before. I think we are all predestined to make certain connections. Me with Chuck and Rikki, Shari with the warriors, and Jeff with Bullitt, all make special connections. How do you advertise or let people know about people who have had TBIs? How does that connect with Shari's desire to create K9 for warriors and how does that connect with Jeff?

There is nothing like that personal soul connection, animal or human. You watch out for each other both physically and emotionally. You instinctively know what the other needs. No words are necessary.

My first "coming back" was when I heard something quietly unzipping by my head on the right side, go up over and down. Then a voice said, "Slowly put your hand out and open it up." I had relearned how to move my fingers, and then my arm on that side, and my mind slowly was able to follow the direction.

When I opened my right eye and hand, Chuck put a couple of small raw carrots in it and Rikki would quietly and easily eat them out of my hand.

Rikki is a golden retriever. When I felt her take it I slowly opened my eyes and I could eventually focus on her. It had taken me quite a while to be able to open my eyes. The right one first and a long time later, open the left one. Then I had to understand that I was seeing something and know what it was.

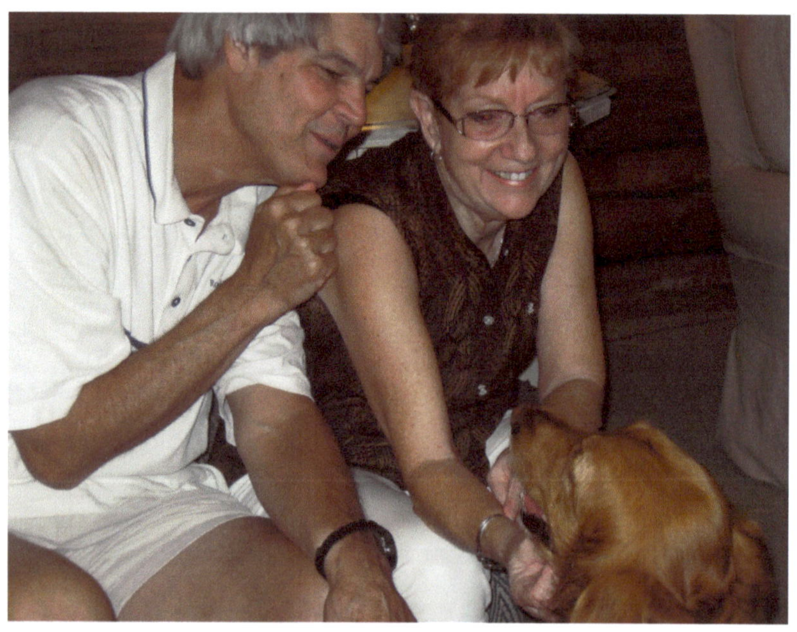

Chuck, Betsy and Rikki

I had had a golden retriever before and maybe it was the first time I had said anything. I said "Lolly". Everybody in the room gasped. Chuck said "no her name is Rikki." Chuck would come in with Rikki

                    Betsy L. Duval

every week and I would immediately wait for Chuck to unzip the tent I was in so he could put the carrots in my hand. Then I could pet Rikki under her chin and connect with her. My dad taught us not to pat a dog who didn't know you on the head. Let it chose to be stroked or it might bite.

I was zipped in the tent on my bed because I had learned to move but my mind hadn't been able to put it all together how things worked. I had emerged off my bed and ended up on the floor one time though somebody, either a family member or friend, was there with me every minute of the day from November 3rd till March 23rd. That was 3 ½ years ago. I was in rehab at Tallahassee Memorial Hospital, Health South, and after that Venice.

For me there is a clear connection for us all. It is easier for us to let ourselves go to a dog. They instinctively know if we are any kind of a threat or if we ourselves are afraid. They don't judge us like some humans do. They even protect us if they know we are afraid and are vulnerable. They become a part of our team.

Two weeks ago Jim and I went to his Brother Bob's home in Ponte Vedra. His wife Shari Duval is the one who originated K9 for warriors. I'll let her tell you her story:

> *Hey Bets. Seems like we both start our days early. Instead of a candle I read my emails, catch up on my Facebook friends and family, and enjoy the quiet time.*

I started K9s five years ago after my Son, Brett Simon, a Canine Police Officer did two tours in Iraq as a bomb dog detector. He and his Bomb dog were placed in some of the most dangerous areas in Iraq with Special Forces looking for Weapons of Mass destruction and weapon supplies. Many of which they found and destroyed. I do not know all that happened to him, he does not talk to Mom about it, but there was death, destruction, and killing. Horror.

When he came home his body was here, but not my Brett, he left that in Iraq somewhere. His smile, his humor, his soul was gone. I did not know him, and as a Mom yourself with your boys you know immediately that something is really, really, bad. I knew this was bad. I did everything I could to bring him out of this dark secret place he chose to go to. He would navigate at night to stores so he did not have to see people, he turned to drugs and alcohol. His demons that he saw, and things they did haunted him. I could not reach inside and pull out the pain, I was helpless. I was watching him self destruct and could not stop it. Finally he got help for the drugs, and we got through that. This was a kid that never drank, and would NEVER do drugs, but he turned to that to "forget" to wipe out the nightmares, the pain. It was after months and months of doing extensive research I stumbled on a new approach for post traumatic stress dis-ability, service dogs. I read everything I could, did my homework, and finally I approached Brett about starting a agency to help Warriors with their PTSD by giving them a service dog. Brett's true gift is the talent and expertise on training dogs,

                     Betsy L. Duval

any dog. It is magic, he is as good as I have ever seen. It is like poetry watching the synergy connection he has with a dog. I could watch it all day, like a fine rider and their horse. It is a talent, a gift.

The LIGHT CAME BACK ON in Brett. I found his switch. The light was not bright, but it was on. Together we worked tirelessly to research, plan and form our non-profit. I was beginning to get my Son back. I am a strong believer that the more you do and give to others, God is pleased and gives you peace and rewards. There is no way I could do this program without God's guidance. He helped us, he guided us through the enormous challenges of starting a non-profit with no money, no resources, but we had determination and a guiding hand.

There was a plan, because what I did not know is there are over 500 thousand other Mothers feeling the same as I did, desperate to help their Sons. Wives trying to help their Husbands.

We worked over a year, and got small donations. Oh a hope, a lot of prayers, and by the Grace of God, challenges, we are where we are today. Brett can turn his experiences to helping others like him, by doing so a little piece comes back every day. He still has his dark days when the demons return, but he will survive, he will flourish, he will raise his Son and be a good Father.

I have my Son Back, and Nothing on earth I am more grateful for.

Love you

Shari Duval

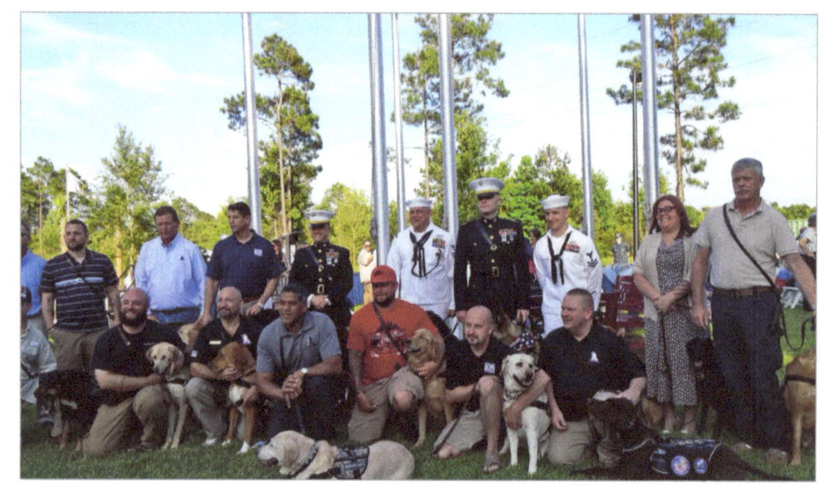

K9s

Every month Jim and I go to a support group for a few hours. It is held in Sarasota but there are centers all over the country. I know I have written to you about this group but hope this gives you a deeper perspective on us. Our special group in the center involves people who have received TBIs. This is definitely a group you don't want to be a part of. We all come together because we are trying to deal with the consequences of our TBIs and how we are going to live with it. At this point we know there is nobody who knows exactly how we feel if it hasn't happened to them. We share with each other our experiences and what has helped us deal with them. We share our positives as well as the negatives.

Bullitt and Jeff are a team. Jeff is part of our TBI support group. His story:

 Betsy L. Duval

My friend from Orlando that has changed my life so much in the last couple of years.... His daughter volunteers for the Orlando animal control. They knew that I was looking for a lab for company, and a therapy and emotional support dog upon the request of my doctor. He knew that I was on the edge of some heavy times (divorce). From what I understand is that a dog came back in for the fourth time and he was ½ Chocolate lab and ½ Doberman. His birthday is July 17, 2012 and needed a home quick. He was to be put down the next morning. Cathie (my friends daughter), found this out and called me and asked me if I would take him. I said yes of course, to give him a try. Within two days, I met Bullitt. I did not know but he was going to be my best friend forever. Since I have had Bullitt from last December he has changed my life if the best way. He not only acts likes me and has my personality, he and myself are best friends. Bullitt watches me all the time and is with me 7/24. He is smart and knows commands which makes him a perfect theory/companion dog. He is licensed and the best thing that I have done in a long time. He has gotten me through the roughest times of my life. The divorce, the selling of the house and splitting up of personal things and being with me while I was setting us up in a new Condo. He has his ways, he loves kids and pretty women. He will wine to them to get attention from them. And he does, they come up to him to pet him and meet me. It is almost like he is setting me up with the right person and not letting me have a say so. Bullitt watches me constantly and I feel very safe with him. We are a pair and I have love him in my heart. This is something that I have forgotten how to do until Bullitt chose me for his companion....

To my best friend, Bullitt...

M. Jeff Vaupel

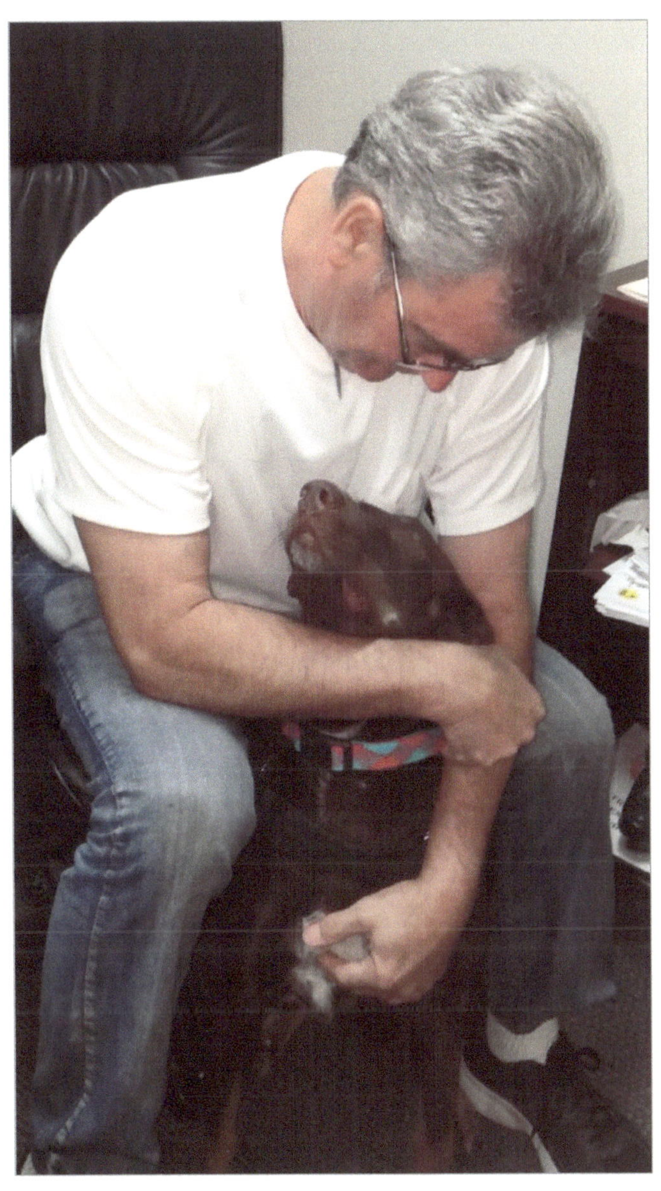

Jeff and Bullitt

Chapter 15

Forward Therapy

My neuro-ophthalmologist referred me to an occupational therapist. She is quite unique. This is a new way to approach people who have received a TBI, stroke or other brain damage. All the doctors are not aware of it or of how significantly it can help one of their patients. Cindy has taken all of her education, licensing, work experiences, physical living locations etc. and now practices her specialty. Her talent deals with how your vision and brain connection affects your overall ability to function. How you hold your head at what angle, how you dodge running into an open door jam, how you step up and down on something, how you walk and balance right, how you reach out and touch something, how far everything is from you, whether it is dark or light, are all connected.

She could tell which of my eyes had more muscle power to keep on target wherever the object moved.

One eye becomes the lazy one when the muscle is damaged with a TBI and recovery has not exercised that eye muscle. In my case there may never be a full recovery but I hope to be able to see slow progress. At least it has the possibility of going forward.

There are exercises she prescribed that I have been doing to help strengthen the inside of my eyeball (the one that was damaged) and help the left one focus with the right one. There is a name for all of that but you and I don't need to remember it. I was excited to know that there was still something I could do to get things more like they use to be.

Presently I think I have gone about as far as I can go with this. It has all improved quite a bit and it has taken me a while to realize and accept that I have done my best. Today is my last appointment with her. I am graduating. She has become a really good friend and cohort both professionally and personally. I'm going to keep up my eye exercises but lately that has been at the top of my list. It will become a part of my life that goes forward.

I am telling you how I became connected with Cindy and her natural talent. This only tells part of her story. She has a degree as a professional. There is no way you could list all the ways and experiences she's had dealing with people with TBIs, strokes, etc. She tells me she learns more every day from her clients. She can even relate more closely now since last month she herself was in a car wreck and feels she might have received a slight damage to her back etc.

At this point I will let Cindy tell you her story. Just stick with your reading. All of us don't have the intellect she does.

Throughout the time I have been going to her I felt she was the one who could help everyone in the support group deal with what they were going through. It all came together last night. It shows what a community of local professionals in their fields, and individuals can receive from each other. She did come to our meeting and it was exciting to see and hear her when she related to them the possibilities that might be available for them to move forward. All exchanged numbers, doctors, needs, access to therapies, etc. It felt good to have been the one to make sure I got them all together. Each of us had had a profession before. Barbara was a registered nurse, Jeff was an electrician, and Ryan was a technician. Now there is no way most of us will be able to make a living wage. Cindy said she feels this is the largest group of under researched or focused on injured people. How do you locate them? How do you get them to come in and get treated? Some of us don't even know we have been injured until it is too late. For an example, we now know that football players who have been knocked unconscious, or somebody who has fallen and hit their head, have all been injured. You might not have come out of it as good as you thought you had. How do you know

            Betsy L. Duval

how to get in contact with them? How can they think about paying for it when they can't work?

There are quite a few of us all around you and you don't realize who we are. Most of us don't look different from the rest of you. We might walk with a slight limp, or have a light tilt of our face to one side to keep our vision focused straight. Never try to judge anybody by looking at them. "You haven't walked a mile in their moccasins". You don't know how good you have it yourself. You are blessed.

I will let her tell you her story:

"My first experience in treating vision deficits after a traumatic brain injury (TBI) was at a special transitional living catastrophic brain injury program out of Texas. I was a young occupational therapist (OT) and had little understanding, the basics of what I learned in text books in college, of treating the vision system and how the visual system significantly impacts all facets of daily function. This original experience was an eye opener, no pun intended. It was also fascinating to treat a patient with severe vision perception deficits, and through repetition, watch the patient improve his ability to interact safely with the environment. Working as a contract therapist, I worked for quite a few great hospital systems after that initial experience and was floored that vision was so often overlooked, under assessed, and certainly undertreated.

The visual system is remarkably complex. It encompasses nearly 70% of the sensory stimula-

tion a person receives at any given time. The other 30% is from the other four senses. Every lobe of the brain, including the brainstem, is involved in vision or visual processing in some way or another. There are over 300 intracortical tracts identified in the brain that relay visual information and often multi-directionally. Vision has far reaching implications and can negatively impact cognition, comprehension of language, posture, balance, gait to just to name a few. It was mind boggling to me that all of the other great rehab programs I worked for did not prioritize assessing and treating vision as a part of the intervention process. If a person is experiencing a visual spatial shift post TBI and that is not formally being addressed, are we maximizing the potential for gait and balance retraining? If a person cannot forecast the next word when reading due to a right homonymous hemianopsia, are we maximizing outcomes with speech therapy and cognitive retraining? It is without question within the OT scope of practice to assess and treat vision deficits that have a negative effect on daily function. So why wasn't this happening?

When I first met Betsy, I was working on developing a vision specific rehab program for neurologically related visual impairments. Betsy was approximately 4 year post her catastrophic TBI and had severe double vision as her eyes really worked independently of one another. She had significant lack of control of her eye muscles. Due to the amazing and inspiring people I have seen progress to independence a year or two post onset of injury, I do not follow the common physician perspective

        Betsy L. Duval

that at 6 months "what you have is what you will have". I believe that due to complexities of the visual system, it lends itself to being highly pliable I nature.

Betsy and I worked to gain better control of her ocular muscles and she worked diligently at home using the simple techniques that I had provided in clinic. The goal was to promote effective binocular function to see a single image at least from 10-20 degrees from center position of gaze. Any movement past that a person will often naturally turn their head so this compensatory strategy would be effective in truly minimizing most if not all of her double vision from a functional perspective. Due to her hard work and determination, we achieved this goal. I should say she achieved this goal. It was amazing to watch this process 4 years post the original injury! My real reward is still hanging in my office and is often used as a talking piece of inspiration for my other patients. It is a copy of the first oil painting that Betsy has been able to complete since her accident. It will always be my reminder that anything is possible".

—Cindy Anderson MHA, OTR/L

Chapter 16

Hugs and HOPE

*W*hich size canvas gets the next "strokes"? Horseshoe, "Evinrude" (dragonfly), bluebird, monarch, southern love knot, dogwood, ladybug, rainbow. It's slowly coming together. "Bling". "HOPE". Right now its home is the back bedroom on the easel. Forward with Hope. Have you seen it somewhere?

We all relate to the atmosphere around us and the conditions we find ourselves in. We are always looking for answers. What do we need to keep us going physically and emotionally? Are we able to extend ourselves out or are we going to draw ourselves in and shut the door so we don't become vulnerable? It takes a lot of courage to step out. "There is a time and place for everything"

Up and out. Still dark. Nothing is up. I quietly slide out of bed. Tap the button on the coffee pot. Pour a cup. Light a candle and the fountain. Water, air, light, and for everything the day comes forward. A bird chirps and another calls back. The sky in the east slowly lights up and I vaguely hear the traffic. Another day. My prayers are answered.

Walk on the beach and pick up a good size conch shell or go to the thrift store or Goodwill and buy a small wine glass or mug. Go to the Dollar Store and get a candle. Put the candle in.

This is your invitation to join our soul group. Your initiation is done with a match. Before the sun comes up, or wherever you are whenever it is, you light it. Surround yourself with peace for the coming day. And know we are all there wishing it for you with hugs and hope. They don't cost anything. Give them to somebody else. They're free. Don't leave it unlit. Share it.

Lv ya!

-Betsy

Additional TBI Resources

TBI Support Group 1-800-992-3442
  www.learningservices.com

Suncoast Center for Independent Living 941-351-9545 www.scil4u.org

Tallahassee Memorial Hospital Rehab Animal Therapy www.tmh.org

Chuck Mitchell www.flcourthousedogs.com www.tmh.org/animaltherapy

TBI Resource and Support www.byyourside.org

Cindy Anderson cynthia-anderson@smh.com

Shari Duval shariduval@K9sforwarriors.org

Dr. Jake Van Landingham jvan@prevacus.com

Service Dogs
  www.assistancedogsinternational.org

VFW Service Dogs swilken@vfw.org

Betsy Duval
  mytbijourney@gmail.com
  jbsjbduval@aol.com

Diane Conti
  Resource Facilitation Coordinator
  Brain Injury Association of Florida
  (941) 800 992-3442
  dconti@biaf.org

TMH TBI Advocacy Group www.tmh.org/TBI